Hilary's Health Haven Handbook

by Hilary Hamilton, CN CHC

Hilary's Health Haven Handbook,

Copyright©2019 by Hilary Hamilton, CN CHC

All rights reserved.

Wildflower Publishing, Lummi Island, WA

Introduction

Welcome to your Health Haven Handbook! I first created this Handbook for myself over the twenty-five plus years of my studying health and nutrition, filling it with the greatest health information to help keep me on track to living my greatest life possible.

I would keep it in my purse for guidance, highlighting and dog-earing the pages, putting my own scribblings in it, and my hope is that you make this handbook your personal own as well.

-Hilary Hamilton

*You can find more of my health writings and favorite recipes on my web-site www.hilaryshealthhaven.com..... You can also find me on Facebook and Instagram under Hilary's Health Haven.....Enjoy!!

Table of Contents

Spiritual Health   119

"You must habit yourself to the dazzle

of the light and of every

moment of your life."

-Walt Whitman

Section One

Emotional Health

Health Practices
for Emotional Wellbeing

Engage in Deep Breathing

Have Morning and Evening Rituals

Move your body daily in an enjoyable way:
put on some music and dance or go for a walk
outside or practice yoga…

Sleep (7-8 hours), Rest and Relax

Engage in Creative Projects

Connect with others who support, nurture, guide
and inspire you

Eat for a healthy Microbiome

Practice Conscious Eating

Watch movies and shows and read books that
inspire you and make you feel good

Watch television sparingly

Listen to Music

Play a Musical Instrument

Sing Songs

Tell your story

Listen to other's stories

Spend time in Silence

Connect with Nature

Spend time with Animals

Participate in a Sound Healing workshop

Practice Aromatherapy with Essential Oils

Create a living space where loved ones can
gather for meals and spend quality time with one
another

Take a Hot Epsom Salt bath

Feel financially rich and abundant by cultivating
gratitude for simple pleasures and possessions.

Practice Self-Nurturance

Practice Self-Compassion

Practice Self-Kindness

Practice Self-Love

Deep Breathing

Forming a deeper awareness of your breath is an important link to optimal health, for when you focus on your breath and use it as a tool, you can create more vitality, energy, balance, healing and calmness, in the mind and in the body.

One great Breathing Exercise to practice for calming and relaxing the body is to sit or lay down in a comfortable position. Exhale out all of your air completely, using the entire ribcage and abdominal muscles to contract in. Then, take a slow inhale for a Count of Five through your nose; during the inhale, your lower belly should expand out first, then your chest. At the end of the inhale, pause for a Count of Two. Then, begin your slow exhale for a Count of Five.

Morning Rituals

Pause, Relax Body, Set Intention for the day

Ask yourself, "What do I need to do to nourish my spirit today?"

Drink water with fresh squeezed Lemon

Drink Green or Herbal Tea

Movement Practice

Meditation

Visualization

Affirmation

Bathe - Self-Care Ritual

Evening Rituals

One hour before sleep - Unwind

Turn off all electronics

Take a bath with epsom salts and lavender

Play soothing music or indulge in silence

Drink a cup of chamomile tea

Read inspirational or spiritual writings

Rub sesame oil on feet

Write in Journal - process out your day, make any lists you need for the future, write five things down that you are grateful for...

Practice Deep Breathing, Visualization, Affirmation and Meditation

Sleep 7-8 hours

"I don't believe people are looking for the meaning of life as much as they are looking for the experience of being alive."

-Joseph Campbell

Practice Conscious Eating

Slow Down

Tap into Intuitive Eating

Enjoy your food

Listen to your body

Eat in a relaxed environment

Breathe deeply

Extend Gratitude

Engage the senses

Chew well and thoroughly
(30 seconds per mouthful)

Observe

Eat for a Healthy Microbiome

It is an amazing fact that there are microbes, which are tiny, single-cell organisms, within our bodies that outnumber our human cells 10 to 1. Each person's microbiome consists of 10 to 100 trillion microbes that primarily live in our guts, but they also live on our skin, and in places like our mouths, nose and genitals. Every individual has a microbiome unique and distinct to them, just like their fingerprint, because the gut microbiome is constantly reacting to the world around and within you.

A healthy community of a variety of microbes within our gut is of the utmost importance because they help to break down food, help sugar and fat metabolism, help absorb vitamins and minerals, help ward off infections, produce B-complex vitamins, and create a strong immune system.

Even more importantly to realize is the fact that this gut bacteria manufactures 95% of the body's supply of serotonin, which is our feel-good neurotransmitters, so a healthy microbiome ensures a healthy supply of feel-good emotions.

One of the best ways to ensure a healthy microbiome is to eat Prebiotic Foods and Probiotic Foods. Prebiotic Foods are the foods that the good bacteria within us love to consume and thrive on. Probiotic Foods are foods that already contain good bacteria that help to re-populate our guts and create a healthy digestive environment.

Top Prebiotic Foods -

The good bacteria in our gut thrive on these foods:

Chicory root

Jerusalem Artichoke

Dandelion Greens

Garlic

Leeks

Onion

Asparagus

Bananas

Walnuts

Pistachios

Top Probiotic Foods -
These foods contain good bacteria that help re-populate your gut

Yogurt

Kefir

Sauerkraut

Kimchi

Tempeh

Miso

Natto

Kombucha

Supplemental Probiotics
(I recommend Dr. Ohhira's Probiotics)

"All that we are

is the result

of what we have thought."

– Buddha

Section Two

Mental Health

"When health is absent,

wisdom cannot reveal itself,

art cannot manifest,

strength cannot fight,

wealth becomes useless,

and intelligence cannot be applied."

-Herophilus

Health Practices
for Mental Wellbeing

Keep a Journal

Stay Curious

Learn new things that engage you and excite you

Engage in meditation to move beyond the
thinking mind

Practice Positive Visualization

Practice Positive Affirmation

"To enjoy good health,

to bring true happiness to one's family,

to bring peace to all,

one must first discipline

and control one's own mind."

-Buddha

Important Questions for Journaling

What am I grateful for?

What is my Intention for my Life?

What is my Life Message?

What gives me strength and inspiration?

What do I most love to do?

What does my future self look like?

How am I allowing myself to play?

How can I simplify more?

How can I listen more?

How can I nurture myself more?

How can I spend more time in silence?

Meditation Practice

One of the purposes of Meditation is to allow a time for you to experience yourself beyond your thinking mind, as someone who is more spacious, open, and full of pure potential.

You can use the breath as the object of your attention while practicing Meditation, which means gently placing your awareness on your breath, feeling and being aware of the breath as it goes in and out.

As thoughts flow into your awareness, just note them, and then gently turn your attention back to your breath, letting the thoughts pass on by, connecting with the open spacious awareness that exists beyond the thoughts.

The Breath can become a steady anchor for grounding and centering yourself, so that at any moment in your life, you have the knowing and practice on how to go beyond your thinking mind and connect with the peaceful spaciousness that exists beyond the thoughts.

The ability to do this will help you make relaxed and clear-headed decisions no matter what is going on in the world around you, and no matter what thoughts are trying to occupy your attention. You will know how to connect with your inner wisdom that knows what is truly best in every situation.

Positive Visualization

With every choice we make and every thought that we think in the present moment, we are creating our future selves.

We can ask ourselves before eating or drinking anything or before taking on any new beliefs, "Will this help me cultivate a healthy future self?"

We can also use our thoughts to create a visualization of our future selves to become a guide for how we live our lives now.

To practice in the co-creation of your future self, you can actively visualize how you want to look and feel in your elder years.

For my own self, I visualize my elder self with beautiful wrinkles on my face that have been created from years of laughing and living in joy.

I visualize how I want to feel, with an energy radiating out from my body that is full of love and compassion and gratitude.

I vision myself continuing to grow and evolve, surrounded by wonderful friendships and community, and being a healing, positive, inspirational force in the world.

What else do you see?

"The golden opportunity you are seeking

is in yourself.

It is not in your environment,

it is not in luck or chance,

or the help of others;

it is in yourself alone."

~Orison Sweet Marden

Positive Affirmations

I am filled with life force energy

I am growing and evolving

I am strong and flexible

I am full of love and gratefulness

I lead a health-inspired life

I am a creative being

I stand in dignity and power

I stand in sacred space

I am boundless potential

All is well in my world

I am a healthy and vibrant being

"To ensure good health:

eat lightly,

breathe deeply,

live moderately,

cultivate cheerfulness,

and maintain an interest in life."

- William Londen

Section Three

Physical Health

Health Practices

for Physical Health

Feed yourself in the healthiest way possible

Understand the best ways to cook beans and grains for easiest digestion

Eat organic, whole plant foods

Have a healthy Grocery List on hand

Have healthy favorite Go-To's and Snacks for eating with greater ease

Eat High Fiber Foods

Eat High-Water Containing Foods for inner hydration and ease of digestion

Be aware of foods that cause the most sensitivity/allergic reactions in people and eat them in moderation, if at all

Be aware of natural anti-inflammatory, anti-biotics, anti-virals and anti-fungal foods and substances for self-healing

Drink pure spring water or use a water filter

Avoid microwaves, use gas to cook

Practice dry body brushing

Get regular monthly massages

Use scrub mitts or hot towel for exfoliation while showering

Use Infrared Saunas

Use Coconut Oil as your body moisturizer in the spring and summer and Sesame Oil in the fall and winter and Argan Oil for your face moisturizer

Take Hot/Cold Showers for Lymph health

Practice body inversions

Use a tongue scraper after brushing teeth

Understand cellular regeneration

Cultivate a healthy lymph

Avoid wearing synthetic clothing, wear natural, organic fiber clothing

Healthy Food Intake Recommendations

MORNING TIME

You will want to go for as long as you can in the morning hours without consuming anything as this allows your body to continue the healing and cleansing process that naturally occurs while you are sleeping....

When you first get thirsty, have a glass of pure water. When thirsty again, have Fresh Lemon squeezed in water. Next, a Green Juice would be fantastic to consume (My favorite juicing ingredients are celery, cucumber and carrot...).

When you feel hungry, a piece of fresh fruit would be excellent as fresh fruit is best eaten on

an empty stomach because fresh fruit is
cleansing, hydrating and quick to digest.

When you feel hungry again, a Green Smoothie
would be a great option as it promotes
consuming leafy greens - blend a nice handful of
kale and spinach and/or leafy green of your
choice with a couple of frozen bananas, enough
almond milk to make it nice and creamy, and a
touch of cinnamon and maple syrup....(a dollop
of sunflower butter and chia seeds is also a nice
addition).

If you want a heartier breakfast, you can have
sliced avocado on toasted sprouted grain bread
with sliced radishes and sea salt sprinkled on

top…You can also just simply have toasted sprouted grain bread with butter.

And one of my absolute favorite breakfast options is a nice bowl of steel cut oats with crushed walnuts and coconut flakes on top, a sprinkle of cinnamon, and a dash of maple syrup.

AFTERNOON AND DINNER TIME

For Lunch and Dinner, always have the major feature of your meal be leafy greens with some diced kale, red and green cabbage, celery, carrots, and fresh herbs (and whatever other vegetables you wish to dice up), drizzled with your favorite salad dressing.

Then, add to this salad whatever other healthy foods that you wish to eat for variety; such as, crushed walnuts, steamed yams, sweet potatoes or small red potatoes, beets, hummus, lentils or black beans, quinoa or millet, guacamole and salsa, steamed or sautéed vegetables, pasta sauce and raw goat cheese, egg omelette with vegetables, or wild salmon....so many yummy combinations to have with your raw salad!

DESSERT

The best option is dark chocolate (70% or above cocoa content)....

For easier digestion, eat simpler meals and follow these guidelines:

1. Eat fruit alone or on an empty stomach

2. Eat grains, beans and potatoes only with other raw or cooked vegetables.

3. Eat any meat dish with only raw or cooked vegetables.

4. Eat nuts and seeds and their butters with raw or cooked vegetables.

5. Try to eat kale and a leafy green salad at least once a day.

'The Rainbow Diet'

Eat the Colors of the Rainbow

Eat at least one food from each of the following color groups every day to ensure you are getting a wide range of phytonutrients. (Phytonutrients are chemicals produced by plants to protect themselves from insect attacks, and in the human body, they have been shown to have anti-oxidant and anti-inflammatory effects.)

GREEN

Brussels Sprouts, Broccoli, Green Cabbage, Kale, Spinach, Leafy Greens, Peas, Beans, Green Bell Pepper, Kiwi, Honeydew Melon, Swiss Chard, Collard Greens, Bok Choy, Artichokes, Asparagus

GREEN/YELLOW

Avocado, Spinach, Mustard Greens, Green
Beans and Collard Greens

ORANGE

Squash, Mangoes, Apricots, Carrots, Pumpkins,
Cantaloupe, Yams

ORANGE/YELLOW

Citrus fruit juices, Grapefruit, Oranges,
Tangerines, Cantaloupe, Peach, Lemons,
Spaghetti Squash, Sweet Potatoes, Pineapples

RED

Tomatoes, Watermelon, Red Cabbage,
Strawberries, Red Bell Pepper

PURPLE/RED

Cherries, Berries, Grapes, Beets, Red Wine,
Raisins

WHITE

Apples, Pears, Bananas, Cauliflower, Cucumber,
Mushroom

WHITE/GREEN

Garlic, Onion, Leeks

Healthiest Foods to Eat

Spinach

Carrots

Blackberries

Asparagus

Kale

Broccoli

Green Peas

Peppers, hot chili green

Strawberries

Brussels Sprouts

Mushrooms, Shiitake

Red Bell Peppers

How to cook 1 cup dried beans

1. Rinse

2. Soak for six hours or overnight (with the exception of split peas and lentils which do not require soaking.)

3. Drain and rinse the beans.

4. Place beans in heavy pot and add 3 to 4 cups of water.

5. Bring to a full boil and skim off foam.

6. Cover and let simmer.

7. Add 1 teaspoon of unrefined sea salt 10 minutes before the end of cooking time.

8. Beans should be tender and soft to squeeze when finished.

Cooking times per 1 cup of dried beans

Black Beans - 60 - 90 minutes

Black-eyed Peas - 60 minutes

Cannellini Beans - 90 - 120 minutes

Chickpeas (garbanzos) - 120 - 180 minutes

Kidney Beans - 60 - 90 minutes

Green Lentils - 25-30 minutes

Red Lentils - 15 minutes

Navy Beans - 60 - 90 minutes

Pinto Beans - 90 minutes

Split Peas - 45 - 60 minutes

Mung Beans - 25 minutes

How to make bean digestion easier:

1. Soak beans for several days.

2. Use a pressure cooker, like the Instapot…

3. Chew beans thoroughly.

4. Avoid feeding legumes to children under 18 months.

5. Experiment with different sizes of beans. Smaller beans like lentils and peas are the easiest to digest.

6. Season cooked beans with sea salt.

7. Add a large strip of dried kombu seaweed to the pot prior to boiling, removing once finished.

8. Add fennel, bay leaves, garlic or cumin during cooking.

9. Add a small amount of apple cider vinegar during cooking.

How to cook Grains

1. Measure the grain, check for bugs or unwanted material, rinse in cold water using a fine mesh strainer.

2. Soak grains for one to eight hours to soften, increase digestion and eliminate phytic acid. Drain grains and discard the soaking water.

3. Add grains to recommended amount of water and bring to a boil.

4. A pinch of sea salt may be added to grains to help the cooking process.

5. Reduce heat, cover, and simmer for the suggested amount of time, without stirring.

6. Chew well and Enjoy!!

Amount of water and cooking time
for 1 cup dried grain

Amaranth	3 cups water	30 minutes
Brown Rice	2 cups water	45 ~ 60 minutes
Buckwheat	2 cup water	20 minutes
Millet	2 cups water	30 minutes
Quinoa	2 cups water	15 ~ 20 minutes
Whole Oats	3 cups water	45 ~ 60 minutes
Wild Rice	4 cups water	60 minutes

Oil Smoke Points

(meaning, if it is a low smoke point, use for salad dressings only and do not heat…)

Low Smoke Point

Walnut Oil

Borage Oil

Evening Primrose Oil

Fish Oil

Flax Oil

Extra Virgin Olive Oil

Medium Smoke Point

Olive Oil

Safflower Oil

Sesame Oil

Sunflower Oil

High Smoke Point

Almond Oil

Avocado Oil

Hazelnut Oil

Macadamia Nut Oil

Coconut Oil

HEALTHY GROCERY LIST

ORGANIC VEGETABLES

Leafy Greens:

Romaine, Baby Lettuces, Spinach, Sprouts,

Swiss Chard, Dandelion Greens, Collard Greens,

Watercress, Arugula, Kale, Turnip Greens,

Mustard Greens

Vegetables:

Broccoli, Cauliflower, Zucchini, Red and Green

Cabbage, Asparagus, Brussels Sprouts, Onion,

Leeks, Mushrooms, Yellow, Green or Red Bell

Pepper, Eggplant, Bok Choy, Garlic, Green

Beans, Celery

Root Vegetables:

Yams, Sweet Potatoes, Small Red Potatoes, Beets, Carrots, Parsnips, Turnips, Spaghetti Squash, Butternut Squash, Delicata Squash, Hubbard Squash, Pumpkin

ORGANIC FRUIT

Fresh Fruit:

Blackberries, Blueberries, Raspberries,

Strawberries, Apples, Oranges, Mangos,

Cantaloupe, Watermelon, Bananas, Pears,

Apricots, Peaches, Kiwi, Lemons, Limes,

Cucumber, Avocado, Olives, Grapefruit,

Cherries, Red and Green Grapes, Tomatoes

Dried Fruit:

Figs, Dates, Apricots, Apples, Pears, Bananas,

Prunes, Goji, Pineapples, Mango

ORGANIC SEEDS AND NUTS

Seeds:

Sunflower Seeds, Sunflower Seed Butter,
Pumpkin Seeds, Pumpkin Seed Butter, Chia
Seeds, Flax Seeds, Hemp Seeds, Sesame Seeds,
Tahini

Nuts:

Almonds, Almond Butter, Almond Flour, Walnuts,
Walnut Butter, Brazil Nuts, Macademians,
Pecans, Pistachios, Cashews, Cashew Butter,
Shredded Coconut, Coconut Flour

ORGANIC GRAINS

Rolled Oats, Millet, Quinoa (Red/White),
Quinoa Noodles, Buckwheat, Soba
(Buckwheat) Noodles, Brown Rice, Brown Rice
Noodles, Basmati Rice, Jasmine Rice, Sprouted
Grain Bread, Kombu, Seaweed Noodles,
Amaranth, Teff, Wild Rice Cakes

ORGANIC LEGUMES AND BEANS

Lentils (Red/Green/Yellow/Black), Mung Beans,
Yellow and Green Split Peas, Black Beans, Pinto
Beans, Garbanzo Beans, Red Beans, Navy
Beans, Adzuki Beans, Kidney Beans, Great
Northern Beans, Cannelini Beans

ORGANIC ANIMAL PRODUCTS

Raw Goat Cheese, Cage Free Organic Eggs,
Raw Goat Yogurt, Fresh Wild Salmon, Organic
Butter

ORGANIC BEVERAGES, etc.

Decaffeinated Organic Water-Pressed Coffee,
Coconut Creamer (for the coffee), Coconut
Milk, Almond Milk, Herbal and Caffeinated Teas:
Chamomile, Peppermint, Dandelion Root Tea,
Yerba Mate, Cinnamon Tea, Green Tea, Nettle
Tea, Rooibus, Carrot Juice

ORGANIC CONDIMENTS

Salad Dressing, Mustard, Tamari Soy Sauce,
Hummus, Guacamole, Salsa, Olive Tapenade,
Marinara Sauce, Mayonnaise, Hot Sauce

ORGANIC HERBS AND SPICES

Rosemary, Mint, Thyme, Parsley, Oregano, Basil, Bay Leaf, Cilantro, Curry Powder, Garam Masala, Paprika, Chipotle, Turmeric, Ginger, Cayenne, Cumin, Coriander, Black Pepper, Cinnamon, Cloves, Garlic Powder, Allspice, Marjoram, Nutmeg, Coriander, Tarragon, Mustard

ORGANIC OTHER

Dark Chocolate, Nutritional Yeast, Coconut Oil, Olive Oil, Sesame Oil, Himalayan Sea Salt, Stevia, Cocoa Powder, Maca Powder, Mesquite Powder, Miso Paste, Green Curry Paste, Spring Roll Rice Paper, Fish Sauce, Maple Syrup, Honey, Molasses, Balsamic Vinaigrette, Apple Cider Vinegar

My Favorite Go-To's for Eating:

~ Green Smoothies: Smoothies are a great way to get nutrient dense foods in a quick way.... Simply blend up a frozen banana or two with some almond milk, and add as many dark green leafy lettuces, kale and/or spinach as you wish.....A large spoonful of sunflower or pumpkin seed butter and chia seeds is also a great addition....

~ Kale Slaw: Place this atop lettuce greens, or as a side for other dishes: diced kale, green cabbage, purple cabbage, sweet onion, beets, carrots, celery, cucumber, bok choy, broccoli and cauliflower.... Then pour on your favorite dressing..... You can also add hummus, guacamole or a simple avocado on

top and mix around.....Add chopped
walnuts for crunch....

- Steamed Vegetables: Vegetables such as
broccoli, cabbage, cauliflower, brussels
sprouts and carrots are great steamed for
5-10 minutes and drizzled with Tamari and
salad dressing....Have these vegetables with
a side of quinoa, black beans or lentils

- Baked Root Vegetables: Set your oven to
450 degrees, and cut an assortment of root
vegetables....beets, yams, small white or red
potatoes, and slices of onion...into steak
fry size.......cook them on Parchment Paper
in the oven for 30-40 minutes....serve with
hummus, black beans, ketchup and salsa...

- Vegetable Wraps: Use either collard greens,
cabbage leaves, or romaine lettuce, as the

'tortilla', spread some avocados and hummus, then add diced bell peppers, tomatoes, red onion, and cucumber, season with a dash of sea salt and pepper, soy sauce and mustard....add pieces of walnuts for some healthy added crunch...

- Vegetable Pasta: Spiralize zucchini, carrots, beets, yams and/or sweet potatoes....Water saute them in a skillet for about 10 minutes until they are soft....Pour a Pasta Sauce that has been cooked with mushrooms, bell peppers, onions, garlic and tomatoes cooked in with it, on top of the spiralized vegetables...Sprinkle on nutritional yeast and chopped walnuts...Serve with leafy greens.....

- Vegetable Soup: Use one part Vegetable Broth and one part Vegetables, bring to a boil, then lower to simmer and cook until vegetables are soft (15 - 20 minutes)… Then, puree the soup ingredients in a blender…The best vegetables to use are broccoli, cauliflower, spinach or carrots….. Season with fresh herbs, spices and miso paste….For thickening, add yams, sweet potatoes or red potatoes and cook for 30 minutes…

- Egg Scrambles: Dice up broccoli, cauliflower, zucchini, tomatoes, mushrooms and onions….water saute them in a skillet for five minutes or until soft, then pour the egg mixture (8 eggs whisked with 1/2 cup Almond Milk) on top of them and scramble….serve with salsa, ketchup and mustard and a side green salad....Add grated goat cheese for added yumminess!

~ Vegetable Sandwich: On toasted sprouted bread, spread hummus and avocado, and then layer lettuce, tomato, onion, slices of bell pepper and fresh herbs on top....then drizzle with mustard, soy sauce and salad dressing for flavor..... (Sliced seasoned tofu is also an excellent addition on this sandwich).

Great Snack Options for Every Day:

- Nuts and Seeds
- Dried figs, dates, pineapples, bananas, mangos, raisons
- Freshly sliced apples, bananas or pears
- Homemade Trail Mix: Mixture of Dried Fruits, Nuts, Coconut flakes and Dark Chocolate nibs
- Bugs on a log: Celery sticks with Almond Butter and Raisins
- Banana with chopped Walnuts sprinkled on top or Almond Butter or Sunflower Butter
- Cut up Carrots
- Cabbage Leaves or Leafy Green Lettuce with Goat Cheese rolled up in the middle with mustard drizzling
- Vegetable Soup
- Coconut or Goat Milk Yogurt

- Black Beans with Salsa and Walnuts

- Lentils and Hummus

- Brown Rice with diced Veggies

- Bowl of Oatmeal with Almond Milk and a touch of Maple Syrup and chopped Walnuts

- Green Smoothie with Sunflower Butter

- Sprouted Grain Toast or Bagel with Organic Butter

- Sprouted Grain Toast or Bagel with Avocado and Sea Salt sprinkled on top

- Sprouted Grain Tortilla Wrap: With Avocado or Hummus or Black Beans, diced Carrots, Tomatoes, Sprouts, and Red Bell Pepper rolled up within it

- Hard Boiled Organic Eggs w/ Sea Salt

- Yam or Sweet Potato Baked Fries, served with Ketchup (Cut Potato Steak Fry Size, put on

Parchment Paper-covered-pizza tray and bake for 30-40 minutes at 450 degrees)

- Quinoa Pasta Salad: Quinoa Pasta noodles or Quinoa mixed with diced sweet red bell pepper, green onion, tomato, zucchini, cucumber, parsley w/ a dressing of lemon juice, extra virgin olive oil, dash of sea salt and black pepper.

High Fiber Foods -

These foods help keep your digestion regular and healthy...

Lentils

Split Peas

Black Beans

Lima Beans

Artichokes

Pears

Avocados

Yams

Peas

Blackberries

Raspberries

Brussels Sprouts

Chia Seeds

Flax Seeds, ground

Chickpeas

Oatmeal

Kale

"Nature, Time, and Patience,

are three great physicians."

~ H. G. Bohn

High Water Containing Foods

(these foods help with satiety and inner

hydration)

Cucumber

Lettuce

Celery

Radishes

Tomatoes

Green Peppers

Watermelon

Apples

Spinach

Star Fruit

Strawberries

Broccoli

Grapefruit

Baby Carrots

Cantaloupe

Pears

Peaches

"Tell me what you eat,

and I will tell you what you are."

-Anthelme Brillat-Savarin

Top Foods that people are usually sensitive or allergic to, so be mindful of consumption and eat these in moderation:

Soy

Gluten

Dairy

Caffeine

Eggs

Nuts

Fish

Shellfish

Sugar!!!

Anti-Inflammatory Foods and Spices

Turmeric

Curry

Garlic

Ginger

Ground Flax Seeds

Chia Seeds

Hemp Seeds

Cherries

Pineapple

Walnuts

Onions

Apple Cider Vinegar

Natural Anti-Virals for viral infections

Apple Cider Vinegar

Oil of Oregano

Garlic

Goldenseal

Oregon Grape

Ginger

Lysine

Lemon Balm

Elderberry

Natural Anti-Biotics for bacterial infections

Manuka Honey

Thyme

Garlic

Oil of Oregano

Cayenne Pepper

Grapefruit Seed Extract

Turmeric

Pau d'Arco

Natural Anti-Fungus for fungal infections

Garlic

Oil of Oregano

Tea Tree Oil

Coconut Oil

Caprylic Acid

Cultivate a Healthy Lymph

The Blood and the Lymph are the two major fluids that run throughout your body, carrying nutrients and oxygen to each and every cell. The Lymph is a colorless fluid that also has the very important role of removing the body's waste products from the body. The Lymph does this by bathing the body's tissues and becoming the medium for the waste that can then be drained from the intercellular spaces to the bloodstream for further removal from the body.

For a healthy and youthful body, it is crucial that this Lymph is able to move easily through the lymphatic pathways, without any congestion or obstruction.

Unlike the Cardiovascular System, which uses the Heart as a pump to keep the Blood moving and circulating, the Lymphatic System does not have an organ designated for pumping. The movement of Lymph depends upon the contraction of the surrounding muscles to move it through the body, so this makes physical body movement a vital key for helping keep the Lymph healthy and flowing.

The physical activity that has been found to be the most effective in moving Lymph is the simple act of jumping up and down vertically. This up and down motion stimulates the millions of one-way valves in the system, as Lymph moves only in one direction through the body's lymphatic vessels. This up and down jumping is best done while jumping on a Rebounder (mini-trampoline), jumping rope or dancing aerobically up and down. At the minimum, you would want to jump every day for at least twenty minutes, building up to more time as you become stronger.

Yoga is also very beneficial for keeping the Lymph clear and flowing, as the tensing and relaxing of the body's muscles while transitioning from pose to pose and then holding the various poses, acts as an internal pump for the Lymph. The Twisting Positions and the Inversions are particularly effective for moving Lymph.

Yoga also incorporates conscious Deep Breathing (pranayama) within it's practice which allows for the lungs to act as the pump for the Lymph. This deep breathing induces a more peaceful and relaxed inner state, which in turn cultivates a more alkalinized inner environment, which the Lymph needs to flow at it's greatest ease.

Lymphatic Massage is also something that can be sought out for helping stimulate Lymph flow and for opening up the lymphatic pathways. During this type of massage, the practitioner uses gentle movements on the surface of the skin where Lymph is located, all in the direction that the Lymph naturally flows in the body.

Dry Skin Brushing also has this same Lymph flow stimulating effect, and it is something that you can do yourself just before getting into the shower. Using a long-handled bath brush with soft, natural-fibre bristles on dry skin, and with long or circular strokes, brush the skin in upward motions from the feet to the torso and then from the fingers to the chest, in the same direction as the Lymph flows, towards the heart. This will also serve as an exfoliating process, removing the dead skin that you are continually shedding every day, thus opening up the pores so that they can breathe more freely.

The Way that you Eat is definitely important in the health of the Lymph fluid, with Fruits and Vegetables being at the top of the list. Those that are Red and Green in color are especially important, such as, berries, cherries, pomegranates, beets and cranberries, dark leafy greens, kale, broccoli and green cabbage. Studies have also shown that one of the main causes of Lymph congestion is the intake of dairy products, meat products and those foods that contain flour and/or gluten, such as breads, cereals, crackers and donuts (etc.). Many people find that when they stop eating these foods they feel much better, with more youthful energy.

Dehydration is another common cause of lymph congestion. The simple act of sipping hot water throughout the day is a great Lymph cleanser, ensuring that there is a pure, flowing fluid flushing it along.

Here are some Amazing Facts about the Human Body's Innate Wisdom and Cellular Regeneration:

1. Each day the body replaces and creates millions of new cells out of the trillion cells in the body.

2. 90% of your atoms are replaced each year.

3. Every 3 to 4 days, the lining of the stomach will regenerate itself.

4. The body sheds more than one million skin cells a day.

5. The surface layer of skin is recycled every two weeks.

6. Between every 300-500 days, the human liver is regenerated.

7. The entire human skeleton is regenerated every ten years or so.

8. About 2 million blood cells die in the human body every second, and the same amount of blood cells are born each second.

9. Every 7 years the body regenerates almost every cell.

10. All of our nails take between 6-10 months to fully regenerate.

With this in mind, you can see that the body has an innate ability to heal and regenerate itself. The cellular structure of the body is not stagnant, but is in a continual process of cellular rejuvenation.

Section Four

Environmental Health

Health Practices
for Environmental Health

Take care of your world by eating a Vegan or Vegetarian diet

Get to know your world environment through traveling to open your mind and know how to eat the healthiest while traveling

Eat organic, and if you cannot, know the Clean 15/Dirty Dozen list of foods

Protect your home by cleaning with the healthiest cleaning products

Use non-harming natural beauty products, natural toothpaste and avoid chemically perfumed cosmetics

Freshen the air in your home by
including green plants

Open a window daily to help circulate fresh air

Understand that there is no separation
between our inner and outer worlds,
so be sure to keep the books you read,
the movies and television programs that you
watch, and the songs and stories that you listen
to healthy and inspiring

Simplify your possessions so that your home
feels organized and calming to you

Live and Eat in accordance with the Seasons

Vegan Food Groups

(to include in your diet every day)

Fruits

Vegetables

Whole Grains

Legumes

Nuts and Seeds

When eating a Vegetarian diet, pay particular attention to getting adequate levels of **Protein, Calcium, Vitamin D, Iron, Zinc and Vitamin B12.**

Here are some helpful lists to help make sure you are getting enough Protein, Vitamins, and Minerals.....

Best Complete Protein Sources for Vegetarians:

Quinoa

Liquid Blue Green Algae

Chlorella

Spirulina

Wheatgrass

Sea Vegetables

Hemp Seeds or Powder

Soy (Organic Only –

Tempeh, Natto and Miso are best)

Eggs

Best Incomplete Protein Sources for Vegetarians:

(Throughout the day, eat a variety of these foods to ensure you get the full amino acid spectrum that makes up a complete protein)

Nuts and Seeds

Beans, Peas and Lentils

Dark, Leafy Greens

Vegetables

Whole Grains

High Calcium Foods

Wild Salmon

Bok Choy

Kale

White Beans

Broccoli

Almonds

Dried Figs

Dark Leafy Greens

Calcium-Fortified Fruit Juice

Sesame Seeds

Seaweed

Raw Goat Cheese

Pumpkin Seeds

Avocado

Butternut Squash

Brazil Nuts

Cabbage

Celery

Asparagus

High Vitamin D Foods

Eggs

Goat cheese

Wild Alaskan Salmon

Fortified Cereals and Beverages

Sundried Shiitake Mushrooms

15-20 minutes of sunlight per day on forearms,

chest or legs also provides your body with

Vitamin D....

(wear a hat to protect the skin on your face

after 5 -10 minutes of direct sunlight, depending

on skin type)....

Most Vegan/Vegetarians do well to supplement

with Vitamin D3....

High Iron Foods

Eggs

Legumes

Dried Dates, Apricots, Berries, and Prunes

Spinach

Pumpkin Seeds

Quinoa

Broccoli

(*Iron is best absorbed when eaten with Vitamin C foods*, such as; Lemon, Lime, Bell Peppers, Kiwi, Oranges, Strawberries, Brussels Sprouts, and Guava)

High Zinc Foods

Wheat Germ

Nuts

Fortified whole grain cereal

Legumes

Pumpkin Seeds

Foods with Vitamin B12

Eggs

Vitamin B12 fortified beverages

Nutritional Yeast

Raw Goat Cheese

*Most all Vegan/Vegetarians should supplement

with Vitamin B12....

Egg Substitutions for Recipes:

1 T chia seeds + 1/4 cup hot Water (Let sit for 5 minutes) = 1 Egg

1 T ground flaxseeds + 3 T hot Water (Let sit for 5 minutes) = 1 Egg

1 T mixed chia/ground flax + 1/4 cup hot Water (let sit for five minutes) = 1 egg

1/4 cup unsweetened applesauce = 1 Egg

1/2 medium ripe banana = 1 Egg

The Best Travel Foods

For Snacking on the road:

Carrots, Nuts and their Nut Butters, Seeds and their Seed Butter, Fresh Fruit (Apples and Bananas), Dried Fruit (Figs, Dates, Prunes, Apples, Bananas, Pears, Raisons), Hard boiled Eggs, Goat Cheese, Hummus and Ak Mak Crackers

For Breakfast on the road:

Fresh fruit

Rolled Oats or Puffed Rice with Cinnamon, Maple Syrup, Walnuts and Almond Milk

Nut butter with a drizzle of honey, or avocado with a sprinkle of sea salt, on sprouted grain bread

Options for Lunch and Dinner on the road -

A One-Pot Meal:

Quinoa or Red Lentils with 2 cups of assorted veggies (such as, diced Carrot, Onion, Kale, Zucchini, Celery, Red and Green Cabbage....)
Season with Soy Sauce, Curry Powder, Ginger Powder, Garlic Powder, Mustard, Ketchup, Veggie Broth, Nutritional Yeast, Turmeric Powder...Put in enough water to cover 1/2 inch and simmer until water is gone...approximately 15 minutes...

Black Beans with diced Vegetables and Salsa

Green Leafy Salad with Yummy Salad Dressing and Crushed Walnuts

Canned Organic Vegetable Soups

Soba or Brown Rice or Black Bean or Red Lentil or Chickpea Noodles, or spiralized zucchini, with Pasta Sauce and diced Vegetables

Smoked Salmon or Goat Cheese with diced kale, celery, carrots and onion, wrapped in a Collard Green or Green Cabbage Leaf as the 'tortilla.'

If you have oven accessibility -

Bake Yams, Winter Squash, Sweet Potatoes, Red Potatoes, Beets, Onions and Garlic Cloves and drizzle with butter

Quick Travel Grocery List

(to be used while traveling with stove-top access...)

fresh apples and bananas and/or dried apples, bananas, figs, dates, prunes, avocados

leafy greens, kale, bok choy, red and green cabbage, celery, carrot, onion, cauliflower, broccoli, yams, sweet potatoes, red potatoes, zucchini, squash

ezekiel bread, oats, quinoa, muesli

black beans, pinto beans, red lentils, hummus, black bean burgers

walnuts, brazil nuts and sunflower butter

butter, cinnamon, chamomile, green tea, dark chocolate, almond milk, salad dressing, miso paste, soy sauce, fruit juice, decaf coffee with half and half, ketchup and mustard, stevia, pasta sauce

eggs

Healthy Restaurant Eating Guide-

Best Choices

Thai/Vietnamese: Summer Rolls, Steamed Dumplings, Thai Papaya Salad/Green Salad, Lemongrass Tom Yum Soup, Lettuce Wraps, Steamed Vegetables, Red or Green Curry

Japanese/Sushi: Miso Soup or Salad, edamame, shumai (mini dumplings), naruto roll wrapped in cucumber rather than rice, oshitoshi (spinach with sesame seeds), salmon tartare, seaweed salad, veggie skewers

Mexican: Tortilla Soup, Vegetarian Tamales, Vegetarian fajitas, Vegetarian Burritos or Enchiladas, Salmon vera cruz, Grilled veggies with black beans and pinto beans

Italian: Minestrone Soup, Pasta e Fagioli, Antipasto, Salad, Salmon

Indian: Mulligatawny Soup, Chana Masala (chickpeas), dal (lentils), vegetable biryani, raita (yogurt sauce)

Middle Eastern/Mediterranean: Israili Salad, Greek Salad with Feta, Olives, Hummus, Veggie Kebabs, Tabbouleh Salad, Foul (Fava Beans), Grilled Salmon

Spanish Tapas: Tortilla Espanola (Egg and Potato Omelet), vegetable paella, marinated mushrooms, white asparagus

SEASONINGS OF THE WORLD

For adding variety and further health to your meals, experiment with International Cuisine Seasonings....

India – ghee (Clarified Butter), garlic, caramelized onions, ginger, chile peppers, cardamom, cinnamon, cloves, coriander, cumin, black pepper, fennel seed, mustard seed, saffron, turmeric, coriander, cilantro, lime, coconut

Eastern/Northern European – pumpkin seed oil, onion, garlic, paprika, caraway, black pepper, allspice, fennel, dill, sorrel, mustard, walnuts

Mexico – lard, garlic, onions, chile peppers, tomato, cinnamon, oregano, cumin, black pepper, cilantro, oregano, marjoram, bay leaf,

lime, cider vinegar, orange, coconut, tomatillos,

pumpkin seeds, peanuts, avocado

Middle East/North Africa/Morocco – olive oil,

garlic, onion, tomato, peppers, saffron,

cardamom, cinnamon, coriander, cloves, cumin,

ground ginger, paprika, fennel, cilantro, mint,

parsley, oregano, dill, honey

Southeast Asia/ Vietnam/ Thailand – sesame oil,

onions, garlic, shallot, chiles, ginger, lemongrass,

lime, cilantro, mint, basil, lime, rice vinegar,

coconut, sesame seeds, peanuts

China – roasted sesame oil, garlic, scallions,

ginger, chiles, cinnamon, cloves, fennel, star

anise, peppercorns, cilantro, rice vinegar, soy sauce, rice wine, honey, fermented black beans

France - butter, olive oil, cream, walnut oil, hazelnut oil, onion, leek, shallot, garlic, tomato, nutmeg, vanilla, saffron, basil, parsley, sage, tarragon, thyme, bay leaf, sorrel, chives, wine vinegar, capers, mustard, wine, cognac,

Japan and Korea- roasted sesame oil, garlic, scallion, ginger, hot pepper, wasabi, rice vinegar, soy sauce, miso, sake, miring (sweetened rice wine), toasted sesame seeds

Italy – olive oil, butter, garlic, onions, tomato, peperoncino, sage, rosemary, basil, oregano, parsley, balsamic vinegar, wine vinegar, lemon juice, anchovies, pine nuts, walnuts

Eastern Mediterranean/Greece ~ olive oil, garlic, onion, tomato, cinnamon, cumin, dill, mint, parsley, oregano, lemon, wine vinegar, yogurt, honey, olives, pistachios, pine nuts, walnuts

The Mediterranean (Southern France, Italy, Spain) ~ olive oil, garlic, onion, tomato, hot or sweet peppers, saffron, fennel seed, thyme, basil, oregano, parsley, savory, rosemary, lemon, orange, wine vinegar, olives, pine nuts, pepperencino, anchovies

The Clean 15

Sweet Corn

Avocados

Pineapples

Cabbage

Onions

Sweet Peas

Papayas

Asparagus

Mangoes

Eggplant

Honeydew Melon

Kiwi

Cantaloupe

Cauliflower

Grapefruit

The Dirty Dozen

(Always buy these Organic….)

Strawberries

Spinach

Kale

Nectarines

Apples

Celery

Grapes

Pears

Cherries

Tomatoes

Peaches

Potatoes

Personal Travel List

(List everything specific to you that you require
for optimal healthy traveling)

Buy Clean Beauty Products that do not have these ingredients:

Methyl-, butyl-, ethyl-, and propylparabens

Sodium laurel sulfate and sodium laureate sulfate

Phthalates

Polyethylene glycol (PEG)

Synthetic fragrances, colors and dyes
Propylene glycol and butylene glycol

Diethanolamine, monoethanolamine, and
triethanolamine

Dioxin

Avobenaone

Triclosan

DMDM hydantoin and imidazolidinyl urea

Use Cleaner Cleaning Products for the Home or make your own:

ALL PURPOSE SCRUB

- 1/2 c baking soda
- Castile liquid soap, enough to make a creamy paste
- 1/2 lemon, to be used as a scrub sponge
- Use damp rag or sponge to wipe away any residue.

ALL PURPOSE CLEANER

- 2 t borax
- 4 T distilled white vinegar
- 4 cups hot water

WINDOW CLEANER

- 1/2 c Castile soap

- 1/4 c distilled white vinegar

- 2 c water

Pour all into spray bottle, shake and spray…
When clean, omit soap and switch to 1/2 c vinegar
mixed with 2 c water to spray and rinse

FLOOR CLEANER

- 1/8 c castile liquid soap

- 1/8 c distilled white vinegar

- 1 gallon water

- 10 drops lavender essential oil

For ceramic and stone floors, eliminate soap and
use 1/4 c vinegar w/ 1 gallon water

Don't use on unsealed wood floors. Instead,
combine 2 c distilled vinegar with 1 T olive oil in a
bucket, let it soak in for 20 minutes, dry mop to
absorb excess liquid.

TOILET BOWL CLEANER

- 2 c water

- 1/4 c liquid castile soap

- 1 T tea tree essential oil

- 10 drop eucalyptus essential oil

MOLD AND MILDEW SPRAY

- 2 cups distilled white vinegar

Put into spray bottle and spray on infected area.

MAKE-UP BRUSH CLEANING

- Shampoo Pea Size liquid glycerin soap and soak in warm water with few drops witch hazel...Rinse Well and Let Dry

Eat in accordance with the Seasons:

Spring ~ Eat more purifying and cleansing foods, such as fresh sprouts, greens and asparagus

Summer ~ Eat more cooling foods, such as fresh salads and fresh fruit

Fall ~ Eat more grounding foods, such as sweet potatoes, yams, beets and onions.

Winter ~ Eat more warming foods, such as veggie soups and baked squash

Live in accordance with the Seasons:

In the Springtime, cleanse your outer environment...simplify and organize...move into action and begin manifesting all that you dreamed and visualized during the wintertime... this is a time of rebirth... a time to put into action new healthier ways of being and seeing.

In the Summertime, rejoice and become present and aware of the warmth and juiciness of this season...enjoy pleasurable experiences...spend time connecting with the earth and the sunshine...

In the Falltime, ground yourself with rituals...this is a time of transformation, a time for practicing in letting go all that no longer serves us...let yourself cry and process out your emotions... strengthen your connection to spirit...rest more and meditate more.

In the Wintertime, spend more time in solitude and silence, in contemplation and prayer...dream and vision and access your deep inner wisdom... Nurture and warm yourself with warm baths, blankets and liquids.

'There is a vitality, a life force, an energy,

a quickening that is translated through you into

action. And because there is only one you in all

time, this expression is unique.

And if you block it, it will never exist through any

other medium….

the world will not have it.

It is not your business to determine how good it

is, nor how valuable, nor how it compares with

other expressions.

It is your business to keep it yours

clearly and directly,

to keep the channel open.'

~ Martha Graham

Section Five

Spiritual Health

"We are not human beings

having a spiritual experience.

We are spiritual beings

having a human experience."

-Pierre Teilhard de Chardin

Health Practices
for Spiritual Health

Be aware of your beliefs, values and ethics

Be aware of your sense of sacredness, wonder
and mystery

See your body as a Sacred Temple

Cultivate time to Pray and sit in Silence

Read Spiritual Writings

Create a Sacred Space for Meditation, Prayer
and Sacred Reading

Practice the Six Paramitas

Cultivate a Spiritual Perspective

Create a Sacred Space

One of the most important relationships that you can cultivate is the relationship that you have with the sacred dimension of life. It is a relationship with the great mystery and intelligence of the universe that is innately infused with love and peace and great meaning. A connection with this sacred dimension can be felt from within you and can be experienced when you intentionally choose to become mindful and aware of its' presence in your life.

A wonderful way to strengthen your relationship with the sacred dimension of life is to create a space within your own home specifically for this purpose. This space will serve as your personal sanctuary; a place where you can go to slow down, become centered, and connected with yourself and the sacred dimension.

You can create this space however feels best for you, making it as big or small as you need it to be. Include within this space the possessions that feel meaningful and inspirational to you;

sacred possessions that help make the space feel like your very own.

You will want to keep this space simple and clean and organized and welcoming to help create a beautiful energetic that you look forward to spending time in.

My own sacred space has a vibrant orange comfortable cushion on the floor, set before a small altar table (the altar was made from a breakfast bed tray table, which I covered with a pretty cloth). On the altar table, I have some of my special stones, gathered sea glass, some crystals, flower petals and pretty leaves that bring nature into the space. I also have a small white candle that I light to bring in the essence of the spiritual. I enjoy having fresh lavender, essential aromatherapy oils or incense there to help cultivate the essence of the space. I have a soft blanket near my altar table to cover my legs and keep me warm and feeling nurtured, and I often bring a cup of herbal tea with me to sip on.

On the altar table, I have images of healthy and inspiring mentors that motivate me to continue growing towards my greatest self, and I have created a Vision Board that holds images of what I aspire to and wish to manifest in my life that I have placed in the center of my space. I also have images of stars and galaxies of the Universe to help remind me to keep a broad and open perspective, and several photographs of my family and my loved ones that warm my heart and bring me joy. There is even a photograph of myself when I was very young, smiling and beaming. These images comfort and nourish me, and make me feel at home in my sacred space.

In this space, I tune in to myself, dropping in to listen and feel what is going on with me. I pick up my journal and begin free flow writing everything that wants and needs to come up. When I feel I have released everything, feeling lighter and more integrated within myself, I then move my awareness to the open spaciousness within me that exists beyond my thoughts that is pure love and peace. I rest there, becoming very close and connected with this space, so that in the future, if I need to, I can drop right in and connect with this love and peace that is always right below all of the chaos.

I also like to read passages from inspiring books that help to motivate and educate my spiritual journey; such as, Julia Cameron's 'An Artist's Way,' a Yoga Philosophy book from Shiva Rea called 'Tending the Heart Fire,' and all of Pema Chodron spiritual books. I keep these inspiring books on a small bookcase that I have in my space, alongside my journals.

My sacred space has provided me a catalyst for discovering my most balanced and centered self. It has also gifted me some of my greatest ideas and insights that have helped guide me on my journey towards greater well-being. And most importantly, it has helped deepen my connection with the love that is always present all around me; whenever I wish to tune into it, it is right there.

Gandhi once said, "Be the change that you wish to see in the world," so if you want a peaceful world, you need to live a peaceful life. I love how the religion of Buddhism maps out six ways of being in the world that will lead to a peaceful and meaningful life, and I try to keep these ways of being in the world in mind as I navigate through the days.

The first is the practice of Meditation where you sit down with yourself as a simple, open, spacious being with pure potential. As you sit there, you put your awareness on your breathing and any time a thought arises, you simply note in your mind, "Release," and then return your awareness to your breath. As you continue to do this, you begin to have an experience of being alive beyond your thinking mind, as a sacred being sitting on sacred ground, and without thoughts to fuel your emotions, you are able to experience a deep sense of peace within you that you can then carry out into the world to share with others. Then, as you move about your day and evening, you can continually return your awareness to your breath and the present moment, becoming an active observer of feelings and emotions, cravings and desires, and simply let them go and return to your sacred, peaceful breathing and life experience.

The second is the practice of Generosity. When you are being generous, you are opening a portal to the deep peace within you because being generous feels so good!! And there are so many wonderful ways to be generous - you can be generous with your time (listening to others, serving others, helping others), with your attention (listening to others, giving affection to others), with your understanding (being compassionate with an open mind), with dropping expectations (which brings great peace to others), with offering wisdom from your own life (sharing your sacred story and personal truth), with creating a safe haven for others (a place that is free from fear and judgement and violence), with not needing to always be right (and instead allowing for peaceful space to reign), with giving someone the benefit of the doubt (and practicing in forgiveness and patience), with being a great health example for others (to inspire others to their own greatest health by sharing health information and giving encouragement). Practicing generosity connects you with an inner energy that uplifts you and others and the entire environment in which you live; it is a complete win-win!!

The third is the practice of Patience which is the antidote to aggression. When you are practicing patience, you are practicing in slowing down, taking a deep breath, opening your mind beyond your thoughts, pausing before you react in a habitual way, connecting with the peace within you and relaxing with the hot energy that feelings and emotions can cause within you. By being patient, you are able to act more wisely with greater thought given before taking any action or speaking any words and you are able to bear witness to the truth that no feeling is final - the hot energy will eventually dissipate and evolve into another inner feeling, opening a portal to a more peaceful inner experience.

The fourth is the practice of Enthusiasm which is a self-cultivated inner energy that helps to fuel your life so that you are able to go forward with an open curiosity and zest for living. Living with a sense of enthusiasm uplifts you and others and the entire environment, just as the practice of generosity does. It is another win-win!! When you foster your own enthusiasm, you are fostering growth, creativity and youthfulness; you are strengthening your inner cheerleader that whispers in your ear all of the positives going on that can help to carry you through any situation. My father is a perfect example of an enthusiastic person who uplifts everyone around him. He was even once at a football game at Penn State where he was a supporter of the visiting football team and he began to get heckled by one Penn State school member saying, "Why did you come here? You are going to get so creamed!" And my father very kindly and enthusiastically responded, "Well, I heard what a beautiful campus you had here and so I was so excited to come here and check it out and it is so beautiful!" And the Penn State heckler just fell silent and looked at him, and the heckler's friends began elbowing the heckler, saying, "Yeah... See! Now, come on and let's go..." And they all just turned and walked away and all that remained was peace.

The fifth practice is Discipline which helps provide us with structure so that we have support and strength for our training in meditation, generosity, patience and enthusiasm. This is the discipline of feeding ourselves in a healthy way, moving our bodies every day, practicing self-love, self-nurturance, self-care and self-compassion.   It is the discipline of remembering to return to gentleness in our speech and actions and thoughts, of seeing the beauty and richness in the simple things of life, of returning to our sacred ground.   It is the discipline of continuing to open to life and not shut down, of clearing the mind to remember that the only thing constant in life is change and transformation.   It is the discipline of remembering to put space in one's life, to slow down and be silent and sacred and spacious, where only pure life aliveness can be experienced beyond all thought as this is where true peace resides.

The sixth practice is Knowledge or Unconditional Wisdom which is the practice of listening to the innate wisdom that lives within us all that knows what is truly the right thing to do in any given situation for the highest good for all. It is the wisdom that is pre-thought, pre-belief and pre-conception. This wisdom tells us that it is best to be flexible and open in one's life, that all is impermanent and changing so every moment is a precious happening that will never happen again in that exact way, and that our human lives are amazingly precious and sacred and should be treated as such. It is the wisdom that cuts through suffering because it sees that all is in process and that all is in perfect order just the way that it is. It is the wisdom that tells you to treat yourself in the healthiest way possible because you are a sacred, spiritual being with many gifts to offer the world. It is the wisdom that tells you that living a life of peace is of the highest order and will bring the greatest meaning to your life and the greatest of happiness. It is a silent, knowing wisdom that leads you on in a gentle, noble way to a life of great integrity and wonder.

These six ways of being in the world are also called the Six Paramitas or the Six Ways of Compassionate Living or the Six Transcendent Activities or the Six Activities of the Servants of Peace. They all mean that these practices will help evolve and uplift and transform your entire life in the greatest of ways. Each practice takes us beyond our own fear of letting go, beyond aversion and attachment, beyond small thinking and small living.

Cultivate a Spiritual Perspective

The earliest pieces of wisdom come from the first human beings ever known to exist - the Aboriginal people of Australia. The Aboriginal's believe that there is a spiritual reality running right alongside the world of day-to-day activities and they called each moment of their lives, 'The Dreaming,' which contained yesterday, today and tomorrow, all wrapped up in one with the sacred spiritual holding them all together.

When you become attuned to this spiritual side of life, an entirely new dimension of reality reveals itself to you...nothing is no longer just black and white, but instead, every happening, no matter how good or bad, becomes a spiritual lesson for you to learn from; for example, you are able to learn your own strength or grow your compassion for those who may be going through the same life situation. And every person you encounter, no matter how good or bad, becomes a spiritual teacher for you, allowing you to practice being open and loving and understanding.

When spiritual consciousness becomes fully functioning in your life, everything that you do becomes an artistry, an intentional placement of action and words for the betterment of all those involved. You become aware of how you can use your own life to beautify the world, to help serve another, to learn the lessons of forgiveness and generosity and love for your own self and for the world around you in a deep and meaningful way. You become more apt to give smiles, hugs, encouraging words, and you evolve to be more of an inspiration to others, which in turn, feeds your own self with more positivity and goodness. It's a complete win-win!

By tuning into the spiritual essence within your own being, you strengthen the sacred in your life and you truly realize that you are so much more than just your thoughts - you are much more open and spacious than that! And your body becomes so much more than just 'a body'; it becomes a sacred temple that houses your spirit and you begin treating it as such - honoring it by feeding your body with nutritious, whole food, and moving it on a daily basis in an enjoyable way that feels good to you.

Joseph Campbell, the famous mythologist, truly knew of the spiritual perspective and explains it when he said, "When you see the Kingdom of the Father (Heaven) spread upon the earth, the old way of living in the world is annihilated. That is the end of the world. The end of the world is not an event to come, it is an event of psychological transformation, of visionary transformation. You see not the world of solid things but a world of radiance.

Your presence in the world is a sacred occurrence and who you are as a human being matters very much to this world - when you shine your loving light and create positivity in another's life, you are making a spiritual difference.

Endnote:

Although this handbook covers the
health essentials, I love discovering and
reading and rereading health
books....here are some of my favorites...
Enjoy!

NATALIA ROSE

- 'The Raw Food Detox Diet'

~ 'Detox for Women'

~ 'Raw Food Life Force Energy'

~ 'The Fresh Energy Cookbook'

KIMBERLY SNYDER

-'The Beauty Detox Solution'

-'The Beauty Detox Power'

-'The Beauty Detox Foods'

-'Radical Beauty' (with Deepak Chopra)

JOEL FUHRMAN

-'Eat to Live'

-'Super Immunity'

GABRIEL COUSENS

-'Conscious Eating'

-'Rainbow Green Live-Food Cuisine'

-'Spiritual Nutrition'

DAVID WOLFE

-'Superfoods'

-'Eating for Beauty'

-'The Sunfood Diet Success System'

ALEJANDRO JUNGER

-'Clean'

-'Clean Gut'

ELSON HAAS

-'Staying Healthy with the Seasons'

-'Staying Healthy with Nutrition'

-'The New Detox Diet'

ANN LOUISE GITTLEMAN

-'Fat Flush for Life'

-'The Fast Track Detox Diet'

-'Super Nutrition for Women'

-'The LIving Beauty Detox Program'

"Everyone has a doctor in him or her;

we just have to help it in it's work.

The natural healing force within each one of us

is the greatest force in getting well.

"Our food should be our medicine. Our
medicine should be our food."

-Hippocrates, The Father of Medicine

Made in the USA
Middletown, DE
13 April 2021